Pegan Diet

Combining Paleo And Vegan Traditions In Pegan
Cooking: A Guide

*(Simple Recipes And A 14-day Meal Plan For A
Healthy Lifestyle)*

Tommie Morrison

TABLE OF CONTENT

What Foods Promote Healthy Digestion?

Eating for gut health is a crucial component of the Pegan diet, as a healthy intestine is essential to overall health and well-being. For optimal gut health on the Pegan diet, consider the following suggestions:

• Prioritize consuming a variety of whole, unprocessed foods, including fruits, vegetables, nuts, seeds, and whole grains. These foods are abundant in fiber, vitamins, minerals, and other nutrients that are beneficial to digestive health.

• Select fermented foods, such as sauerkraut, kimchi, and yogurt, as they encourage the development of healthy bacteria in the gut.

• Steer clear of processed and refined foods as well as those high in added sugars, sodium, and unhealthy lipids. These foods may be detrimental to your digestive health and may disrupt the balance of beneficial bacteria.

• Be aware of your body's response to various foods and beverages, and pay attention to your body's signals. Consider how you feel after consuming and drinking, and avoid foods and beverages that cause digestive issues or discomfort.

• Consult a healthcare professional or registered dietitian if you are concerned about your gastrointestinal health or if you are experiencing digestive issues. They can offer customized guidance and assistance on how to consume for optimal gut health.

It is essential to note that the Pegan diet is an individualized dietary plan, and that health guidelines may vary based on your personal preferences and health objectives. If you are uncertain about how to follow the Pegan diet, or if you have concerns about your health, it is best to consult with a healthcare provider or registered dietician who can offer personalized advice and support.

CHAPITRE SEVENTEEN

What foods promote longevity? Eating for longevity is a crucial component of the Pegan diet, as a healthy diet can promote excellent health and well-being throughout the lifespan. • Select foods high in antioxidants, such as berries, dark leafy greens, and fatty fish, as these can help defend against chronic diseases and promote healthy aging.

SECTION SEVENTEEN

What foods improve mood? Eating to improve mood is an essential component of a healthy diet, as the foods we consume can have a substantial effect on our mental health and well-being. • Choose foods that are rich in omega-3 fatty acids, such as fatty fish, flax seeds, and chia seeds, as these can help to enhance mood and reduce depression and anxiety symptoms.

EIGHTEEN

Make healthy dining affordable

There are methods to make healthy eating more affordable, despite the perception that a healthy diet can be expensive. The following suggestions can help make healthy dining more affordable:

• Plan your meals ahead of time and create a purchasing list to save money and avoid impulse purchases.

• When fruits, vegetables, nuts, and whole grains are on sale, store up.

• Consider buying in volume, as this may be more cost-effective than purchasing food in smaller quantities.

Utilize coupons and loyalty programs to save money on nutritious foods.

• If feasible, grow your own fruits and vegetables to save money and ensure that they are fresh and organic.

• Use seasonal fruits and vegetables because they are typically less expensive and more flavorful than out-of-season produce.

It is essential to note that the cost of healthful eating can vary based on location, personal preferences, and dietary requirements. You can make healthful eating more affordable and accessible for your family if you plan ahead and shop wisely.

NINETEEN

Feed your children what you eat

On the Pegan diet, it is essential that you feed your children the same foods that you consume, as this ensures that they receive all the nutrients necessary for their growth and development. The Pegan diet focuses on whole, unprocessed foods, such as fruits, vegetables, nuts, seeds, and whole grains, which are nutrient-dense and can promote excellent health. By consuming the same foods as your children, you can serve as a role model for healthful eating and assist them in developing a positive relationship with food.

SECTION TWENTY

How do you maintain healthful eating habits?

It can be difficult to maintain healthy eating habits, but there are methods to increase your odds of success on the Pegan diet. To maintain healthy eating habits on the Pegan diet, consider the following suggestions:

• Start small and make gradual adjustments to your diet, rather than attempting a complete overhaul of your eating habits. This may facilitate an easier and more manageable transition to a healthy diet.

• Prepare nutritious snacks, such as chopped fruits and vegetables, to have on hand for when you are hungry. This can prevent you from consuming toxic foods and beverages.

• Be aware of your eating habits and how you feel after you consume. This can help you identify hazardous patterns and make dietary adjustments.

• Maintain a food journal or utilize a tracking application to track your eating behaviors and identify areas for improvement.

• Find healthy alternatives to your favorite unhealthy foods, such as substituting avocado or hummus for mayonnaise as a condiment. This will allow you to appreciate your favorite foods without sacrificing your health.

Noting that establishing healthy dietary habits can take time, effort, and possibly trial and error is essential. You can establish healthy eating habits that support your health and well-being on the Pegan diet by being consistent and persistent.

SECTION TWENTY-ONE

Start the vegan diet immediately The Pegan diet provides numerous health benefits, such as weight loss, decreased inflammation, enhanced gut health, and increased energy. In avoiding processed and refined foods and emphasizing plant-based foods that require less water, land, and energy to produce, it is also a sustainable and environmentally-friendly way of consuming.

If you are interested in beginning the Pegan regimen, here are some guidelines to help you get started:

• Consult a healthcare provider or registered dietitian to determine if the Pegan diet is appropriate for you based on your medical history, nutritional requirements, and health objectives.

• Educate yourself on the principles of the Pegan diet and become familiar with the foods and beverages that are permitted and those that are not.

• Develop a strategy for incorporating the Pegan diet into your lifestyle, including meal planning, grocery purchasing, and food preparation.

• Adopt the Pegan diet gradually and give yourself time to adjust to the new method of eating.

• Consider your body's reaction to the Pegan diet, and pay attention to its signals. If you experience any adverse effects, such as vertigo, fatigue, or digestive issues, discontinue the diet and consult a physician or registered dietitian.

The Pegan diet is a nutritious, eco-friendly, and delectable eating plan that can support your health and vitality.

TWENTY-TWO

Cook according to the pegan method To cook Pegan-style, you can follow these guidelines:

• Utilize whole, unprocessed ingredients, including fruits, vegetables, nuts, seeds, and whole cereals. These ingredients are the basis of the Pegan diet and provide a variety of nutrients and health benefits.

• Select culinary methods that maintain the nutritional value of the ingredients, such as steaming, boiling, grilling, roasting, or baking. These cooking techniques can add excess fat and calories to your food.

• Use healthful fats for cooking and seasoning, such as olive oil, avocado oil, and coconut oil. These fats, such as hydrogenated oils and Tran's fats, are detrimental to your health and should be avoided.

• Experiment with various herbs, spices, and seasonings to add variety and flavor to your dishes. Avoid condiments that have been processed, such as ketchup and mustard, as they are often high in sugar and sodium.

• Prepare nutritious snacks, such as chopped fruits and vegetables, to have on hand for when you are hungry. This can prevent you from consuming toxic foods and beverages.

By adhering to these guidelines, you can prepare delectable and nutritious meals that adhere to the Pegan diet's tenets.

Here Are Some Suggestions For Vegan Breakfasts

Blend together rolled oats, almond milk, chia seeds, and your preferred fruit, such as berries or bananas. Refrigerate the mixture overnight, and savor it in the morning with a sprinkle of nuts or seeds for added texture.

Eggs scrambled with vegetables:

In a skillet, scramble eggs with your preferred vegetables, such as bell peppers, shallots, spinach, or tomatoes. For a scrumptious and nutritious breakfast, serve the eggs with a side of avocado or whole grain toast.

Smoothie glass:

Fruit, such as berries, avocados, or mango, is blended with almond milk, spinach, and chia seeds. Pour the smoothie into a bowl and garnish it with nuts, seeds, coconut flakes, or granola, as desired.

SOUPS AND SALADS.

Here are some suggestions for vegan dishes and salads:

To make tomato soup, bake cherry tomatoes with garlic, olive oil, and seasonings until soft and caramelized. Blend the tomatoes with vegetable broth in a blender, then season the soup to taste with salt and pepper. Serve the broth drizzled with olive oil and garnished with fresh herbs. To prepare lentil soup, sauté onions, carrots, and celery in olive oil until tender. Add lentils, vegetable broth, and herbs and seasonings of your choosing, such as cumin and coriander. Soup should be simmered for approximately 30 minutes, or until the legumes are tender. Serve the broth with whole grain bread or a small salad on the side.

Mix romaine lettuce with sliced chicken breast, cherry tomatoes, and croutons for a Caesar salad. Blend avocado, garlic, lemon juice, and olive oil in a food processor or blender, then season with salt and pepper to taste. Toss the salad with the vinaigrette and garnish with Parmesan cheese or nuts for additional flavor and texture.

Cook quinoa in simmering water according to the instructions on the package. Combine quinoa, cucumber, cherry tomatoes, and parsley. Make a vinaigrette by combining olive oil, lemon juice, and garlic, then seasoning it to taste with salt and pepper. For added protein, toss the salad with the vinaigrette and serve with grilled chicken or salmon.

In a large basin, combine chopped lettuce, bell peppers, carrots, onions, and avocado. Add flavor and nutrition to the salad by topping it with seared chicken or salmon, for example.

This minced salad is a healthy and satisfying lunch or dinner option for vegans. It is nutrient-dense and readily adaptable to individual preferences and dietary requirements.

What Can You Eat?

When it comes to sticking to a diet, the majority of us struggle with the same issue: how do we begin? While the majority of people can readily identify what to consume, the primary issue is that individuals lack the motivation to acquire.

begun. If you wish to begin a vegan diet, you can do so by adhering to the following guidelines.

1. Is the sustenance natural (created by God) or man-made?

Regardless of the sort of diet you follow, there is only one rule you must adhere to: consume actual foods and not food-like substances. Actual foods are those without labels, which may also contain constituents you can pronounce and identify. This variety of food undergoes little transformation from field to plate.

2. Attempt to avoid purchasing foods with numerous labels. You must avoid consuming foods with labels. If the ingredients used in these dishes are those you would typically find in your kitchen, they are acceptable.

In addition, you should avoid goods with health and wellness claims on the labels. Only refined food-like substances have labels such as 'Heart-Healthy' and 'All-Natural. These labels will never appear on a container of broccoli or kale. These health claims are intended to deceive consumers. As an illustration, gluten-free potato crisps are unhealthy. Actually, you do not need a health claim to recognize that whole vegetables and fruits are beneficial to your health.

3. Avoid ingredients that you cannot pronounce or that you would not maintain in the kitchen.

Why would you purchase foods that contain artificial sweeteners, MSG, dyes, chemicals, and other substances that you would not normally keep in your home?

You should never ingest foods that contain ingredients you cannot even pronounce. Avoid eating GMO ingredients. 4. Always explore the outer aisles of the grocery store. Professionals recommend shopping around the perimeter of a supermarket. By doing so, you will recognize that you are purchasing authentic foods. This is the location where you can find fresh foods such as fish, eggs, poultry, meat, fruits, and vegetables.

Typically, processed food-like materials are located in the central aisles. Check the exterior aisles frequently for the finest health foods. The only exceptions are oils, seeds, and legumes that are ordinarily found between aisles.

5. Consume primarily plant-based diets.

It has been clinically demonstrated that plant-based diets contain a variety of disease-fighting and beneficial substances. When preparing a dish, you should always aim to fill 75% of the plate (by volume) with plant-based foods. Consume always vegetables such as kale, peppers, tomatoes, arugula, bok choy, and broccoli. If you have prediabetes or diabetes, you should avoid starchy vegetables. You can also consume fruits with a low glycemic index, such as citrus and berries.

6. Meat is used as a condiment and not as a main component of the dish. While flesh is permitted on a vegan diet, it is not the primary focus. All you need on your dish is a palm-sized amount of

protein, which is roughly equal to one ounce.

consists of both plant-based and animal proteins. Always search for fatty fish, pasture-raised eggs or poultry, and grass-fed meat when following a pegan diet. Alternately, you can search out organic and non-GMO tempeh or tofu.

The vegetables should be the centerpiece of your tray, and the meat should be the side dish. It is recommended that you consume 4-6 ounces of animal protein per day.

When referring to sugar in this context, we do not mean beet sugar; rather, we are referring to walking stick sugar. Vitamins and minerals are extracted from the carbohydrates in sugar cane to create molasses; the remaining substance is white sugar. If you want to overcome your sugar cravings, you must work with insulin and maintain stable blood sugar levels. If you want to decrease sugar cravings, you must eliminate carbohydrates and grains from your diet. You can search for high-quality chromium supplements online and also take them with your meals in order to stabilize your blood sugar levels and also reduce your sugar cravings.

7. ingest fat

As we already know, fat is essential for the proper functioning of the human body. It is one of the most basic building elements. Typically, a person consists of 15-30% fat. Contrary to erroneous information, healthy and balanced fats are required for healthy fertility, brain function, cells, and epidermis.

Unhealthy lipids, such as refined vegetable oils, are harmful to health and wellness. Always consume three to five servings of healthful fats, such as olive oil, seeds, nuts, and avocados. A single serving of fat consists of one-half of an avocado or one teaspoon of olive oil.

8. Include unique superfoods.

The term "superfoods" can be applied to any food that is nutritionally dense to the brim. This article has repeatedly mentioned fatty salmon, grass-fed meat, and plant-based foods as examples of superfoods that you should consume on a daily basis. 9. Consider low-starch legumes, seeds, and nuts.

Seeds and nuts are mainstays in a standard vegan diet. In addition to being an excellent source of minerals, protein, and fiber, beans can also cause digestive issues. If you are diabetic, a diet consisting primarily of beans can cause serious problems with your blood sugar levels. If you have an autoimmune disease and/or insulin resistance, you may benefit from a temporary bean-free diet.

It is recommended that you consume low-starch legumes such as lentils, lupine beans, and black beans. Seeds and legumes are two of the most popular superfoods.

You can incorporate seeds and nuts such as hemp seeds, macadamia nuts, chia seeds, and almonds into your daily diet.

10. Avoid the vast majority of dairy products.

The majority of paleo and vegan diets discourage dairy consumption. It is known to cause a variety of complications, including osteoporosis, cardiovascular disease, diabetes, sinusitis, obesity, and acne. If you enjoy milk products, look for those that are high in nutrients, such as cheese, goat/sheep yogurt, clarified butter, and butter.

11. Always choose whole cereals.

Granted, we do not require grains for food, but this does not imply that they conduct badly for us. If consumed in the form of flours (read more: white flour), blood sugar levels can increase. Daily avoidance of flour-based gluten and gluten-containing products is required. Gluten cereals such as heirloom rye, einkorn wheat, and barley can be consumed if you are not gluten-sensitive. However, specialists recommend a three-week gluten-free evaluation. Later, you can reintroduce gluten to determine its effects. Once you realize how much healthier a gluten-free diet is, you will certainly appreciate this. There are exceptions, such as almond flour. You must avoid flours derived from grains. Always include small portions of low-glycemic cereals, such as quinoa and black rice. If you have an autoimmune disorder, abdominal obesity, insulin resistance, or if you are pre-diabetic or diabetic, eliminate grains completely for three weeks and then assess how you feel. 12. Consume indulgent foods, but not every day.

A pegan diet is not about perfection; eventually, we may deviate from this daily routine and indulge in some delicious fast food or processed foods. The primary objective here is to prevent these minor indulgences from becoming full-fledged habits. You can also occasionally appreciate saccharine.

Instead, choose these indulgences occasionally while adhering to your vegan diet 90% of the time. If you have a craving for French fries, you can create them yourself using salt and truffle oil; as a result, you will be able to munch on delicious and straightforward french fries. You can enjoy a mixed cocktail or red wine with your friends once every few weeks or months. You must ensure that the occasional indulgences you consume are real, whole foods and not the food-like substances we have previously discussed.

From the foregoing, it is clear that a vegan diet will help restore your health and the health of the entire planet. A pegan diet is comprised of these simple principles, which are personalized based on daily needs. Top Superfoods to Include in Your Diet The concept of food as medicine is regarded as one of the most potent tools or ideas for achieving optimal health that you have presented. In addition, using food as medicine should be the initial action you take to treat chronic health conditions of various types. While there are numerous varieties of nutrients on the market today, they can all be separated into distinct categories. In this section, we will discuss the following categories of superfoods:

1. Seeds

There are primarily three types of seeds that you must take into account: hemp, chia, and flax. The chia kernel is a

They are an excellent source of omega-3 fatty acids and contain more calcium than milk. Furthermore, they are an

They are an excellent source of anti-inflammatory substances, making them ideal for attractive skin, mental health, and much more.

A single ounce of chia seeds contains approximately 10 grams of fiber; additionally, the fiber in chia seeds is an insoluble fiber that feeds the gut-friendly bacteria, which promotes digestive tract health and also ferments into short-chain fats that are extremely important for intestine health. In addition to being an exceptional source of healthy proteins, chia seeds contain more protein than most plants.

In addition to being an excellent source of fat, hemp seeds are rich in Vitamin B, nutritious protein, magnesium, zinc, and iron. Additionally, flax seeds are rich in omega-3 fatty acids, dietary fiber, essential vitamins, and minerals. They also contain lignans, which are potent hormone-balancing anti-cancer agents. Experts recommend that you include ground flax seeds in your smoothies to support when you are pregnant or breastfeeding.

are experiencing problems based on

irregularity. Healthy bowel function.

2. MCT oil

Medium-chain triglyceride (MCT) oil is a type of fatty acid derived from coconut oil. MCT oil is a type of superfuel for your cells because it promotes fat metabolism and also improves mental performance. MCT oil aides in weight loss due to the rapid rate at which it is burned and metabolized. Additionally, the oil is absorbed directly from the gut into the liver, where it is not retained as fat and is rapidly converted to energy. MCT oil can be added directly to smoothies, coffee, salad dressings, etc.

3. Glucomannan

From the foregoing, it is clear that you need fiber in your diet to maintain health and balance, as well as to provide sustenance for the healthy bacteria in your digestive tract. As gatherers and hunters, humans once consumed approximately 150 grams of fiber per day, compared to 20 grams today. Fiber is known to prevent obesity and all other chronic diseases associated with aging. This is due to the fact that fiber delays the rate at which food enters the bloodstream and also increases the rate at which food leaves the body via the digestive system. Fiber maintains a healthy balance of blood glucose and cholesterol, eliminates toxins from the body, and reduces appetite.

It is derived from the cognac root, also known as the elephant yam. The cognac tuber has been used for centuries as an organic ingredient in the production of conventional foods such as brandy jelly vermicelli and tofu.

One of the finest ways to consume glucomannan is through a supplement known as PGX. Numerous studies have been conducted on topics such as fat metabolism, diabetes, cholesterol, etc. PGX can be added to water daily and is a simple and dependable source of potassium.

fiber.

4. Mushrooms

When discussing mushrooms, we are not referring to a single species, but rather all of them.

comprehensive category of food. It is fascinating to learn that the average Chinese person is more knowledgeable about the medicinal properties of food than many western researchers and scientists. This is due to the fact that medical goods are part of their daily diet.

Mushrooms such as cordyceps, maitake, shiitake, reishi, etc. are a fundamental part of the Chinese diet. All of these mushroom varieties have powerful restorative properties that can boost your immune system and support your hormones.

In addition, they are anti-viral, anti-inflammatory, and antibacterial.

Additionally assist in liver recovery. Mushrooms can also reduce cholesterol levels. You can prepare reishi tea or shitake mushrooms for soups.

5. Plant nutrients

Yes, the extensive array of colors in vegetables represents approximately 25,000 compounds and chemicals that are extraordinarily beneficial to the body.

- They are referred to as phytochemicals. There is some evidence that the interaction between colors confers additional benefits, so it is recommended that you consume the rainbow. You must have a variegated diet and consume a variety of colored fruits and vegetables.

Vegetables and fruits are historically and inherently essential. Our ancestors, the hunters and gatherers, ate over 800 plant sustenance varieties. We do not consume nearly as much as we did in the past.

We must exert additional effort to increase the variety of our daily diets.

Always according to experts, you should consume the colors of the rainbow. This is because each color of fruits and vegetables represents an entirely different family of recuperative compounds. Red vegetables and fruits such as tomatoes contain the carotenoid lycopene, which aids in the elimination of cancerous cells.

Free radicals that are known to damage our genomes and prevent various cancers, including prostate cancer.

cancer.

In contrast, green vegetables and fruits contain compounds such as isocyanates, indels, and Fleur Fane, all of which help prevent cancer cells by inhibiting health risks and eliminating them from the body.

It is necessary to attempt them all, including purple, yellow, orange, white, blue, etc. All of these vegetables and fruits have remarkable benefits.

To prevent access to this section, experts recommend taking your medications daily. Consumption of these superfoods is always the superior option. Always remember that these nutrients are more powerful than anything you will ever find in a prescription bottle.

The Pegan Diet

If you're contemplating going Pegan, you're thinking wisely, my friend, because going Pegan implies going clean, going new, and going gracious so scrumptiously good. Pegan is the joyful combination of the Paleo and Vegan diets.

The Paleo lifestyle is a return to consuming the way our ancestors did thousands of years ago. Clearly, our Paleolithic ancestors did not consume Twinkies and microwave pizzas, as processed food varieties are a relatively recent invention due to modern machinery.

Before processed food, banquets required scavenging the land and consuming fire-cooked or crude foods. The average diet would have consisted of natural products, vegetables, legumes, and animal protein.

The remaining portion of the Pegan lifestyle consists of Vegan diet components. Vegetarians do not consume large quantities of animal proteins or animal products like yogurt and eggs. In all other respects, their diet consists primarily of pure, whole food sources, such as fruits, vegetables, nuts, and grains.

These foods will keep you healthy, satiated, and radiant. Have pink grapefruit with Coconut Lime Dressing for an exquisite cell-reinforcing breakfast boost in the morning, or perhaps Coconut Pancakes with Peaches and Walnuts for a debauched informal Sunday breakfast.

The lunch contributions are delectable, if I may say so myself. Try the Pistachio

Jewel Salad or the Hearty Cabbage and Fennel Soup for a taste of the unfamiliar.

When the dinner bell rings, fire up the grill and serve Portabella Mushroom Salad with Almond Honey Cauli-Skewers as an appetizer. And you will not need to forego dessert, as the offerings are substantial and incredibly delectable, such as our signature Strawberry Cashew Cake.

Differences among Paleo, Pegan, and Vegan Diets

The Pegan diet is achieved by combining Paleo and Vegan principles. Paleo standards require adherents to consume only natural meats, poultry, seafood, organic products, vegetables, nuts, and seeds. In addition to grains, vegetables, and processed foods, dairy products are prohibited on the Paleo Diet.

For the vegetarian diet, adherents may consume fruits, vegetables, nuts, and seeds while eliminating all animal proteins, such as those found in milk and cheese.

When combining the Paleo and Vegan dietary universes, the resulting table of food options is particularly robust. On the Pegan diet, it is permissible to consume a broad variety of fruits, vegetables, nuts, and seeds (similar to the Vegan diet), as well as a limited amount of animal protein.

In contrast to the Paleo diet, which eliminates all grains and vegetables, the Pegan diet allows for limited amounts of these foods each day.

Pegan Guidelines

Fruits, Veggies

Fresh vegetables and natural products are always fashionable on the vegan diet.

You can consume large quantities of raw or prepared vegetables, and fruits are also a healthy option. However, you should limit your consumption of high-sugar fruits, such as pineapple, because an excessive amount of sugar is unhealthy.

 Seeds and Nuts

Nuts and seeds are rich in heart-healthy lipids and would have been an integral part of the Paleolithic diet. Consuming a small amount of nuts and seeds daily will keep you satiated and provide you with the essential fats for healthy skin, hair, and nails. However, keep in mind that it's easy to consume a large amount of nuts and seeds, and despite the fact that it may appear that you've only consumed a small amount, nuts contain a high amount of fat in a single small nut. When consuming almonds, observe portion control.

Animal-Based Goods

Now that animal proteins are permitted on the Pegan diet, think of them in the same way you would think of sprinkling parsley on a dish; that is, the animal protein is not the main attraction on your plate, but rather an embellishment or a seasoning. Additionally, when selecting poultry, meats, and fish, ensure that they have been grain-fed or are untamed, respectively.

Eggs

The Pegan diet recommends consuming two eggs per day for protein and to ensure satiety, so that you do not feel compelled to consume unhealthy foods.

Grains and Legumes

The Paleo diet eliminates all grains and vegetables, whereas the Pegan diet allows you to incorporate small portions of both into your daily diet. Consistently consuming a half-cup of low-glycemic grains such as quinoa is recommended for satiety. Additionally, you can consume up to half a cup of vegetables daily for a protein boost.

The Pegan Distinction

Eating the Pegan way entails adopting healthy eating practices and consuming nutrient-dense, perfectly prepared, and delicious food. It is a well-balanced diet that ensures adequate intake of essential nutrients, from proteins to carbohydrates.

Eating the kinds of foods that your body enjoys also means that your body is better able to process them and convert them into the nutrient-rich fuel it needs to remain healthy, happy, and energized.

The Pegan Diet

The Pegan Diet is a prominent global diet that originated from an illogical combination of the Paleo and Vegan diets. Pegan was created by Dr. Mark Hyman, the director of the Cleveland Clinic Centre for Functional Medicine, who claims that the Pegan diet is the most rational and healthful diet ever devised for humans.

The Pegan Diet, devised by Dr. Mark Hyman, is a combination of the paleo and vegan diets, founded on the premise that both paleo and vegan eating (when practiced correctly) emphasize the consumption of whole, fresh plant foods.

Dr. Hyman has assisted countless men and women around the world in losing weight, repairing their digestive systems, managing difficult conditions such as depression and anxiety, and even reversing life-threatening diseases such as type 2 diabetes, high blood pressure, and cancer.

To comprehend the convergence, one must first examine the numerous involved elements:

1.1 The Vegan Diet

The most essential aspect of a vegan diet is avoiding animal products and focusing on plant-based foods. This diet lacks meat and other biomolecule-rich foods, including dairy and eggs. The majority of vegans are quite choosy eaters. In addition to the restrictions outlined above, they avoid processed animal ingredients like gelatin, which is frequently added to dishes, even those that appear vegan.

The result is a low-calorie, low-cholesterol, and low-saturated fat diet. As it regulates cholesterol and blood pressure, it is also beneficial for cardiac problems. Veganism is gaining popularity due to its numerous health benefits.

Veganism has numerous health benefits, including a reduced risk of obesity, certain cancers, and type 2 diabetes.

However, the diet is deficient in certain amino acids, which are the building elements of protein and can only be obtained through food. In addition, it is lacking in iron, calcium, zinc, and vitamin B12.

1.2 Paleolithic Diet

Its adherents were the ancient inhabitants of the Stone Age. As with its antecedents, the Paleo diet relies solely on foods available to your ancestors and excludes or restricts modern foods. The paleo diet emphasizes meat and vegetables, with a small amount of fruits and legumes for variety. As additions and replacements, grains, legumes, added sugar, dairy, and a variety of oils should be avoided.

In contrast, your hunter ancestors ate grass-fed meat, seafood, eggs, nuts, fruit, and organic low-starch vegetables, as did the cave people, the creators of the paleo diet. Cereals, legumes, refined sugar, potatoes, the majority of dairy products, and certain oils are prohibited despite the fact that their fat content is not regulated.

The majority of Paleo dieters consume minuscule portions of meat at each meal. It suggests that meat contributes between 30 and 50 percent of daily energy. Compared to current dietary guidelines, which recommend that meat should comprise 15% to 25% of daily calories, these quantities are twice as high.

1.3 The "Pegan" Diet

Following a set of guidelines when developing a diet plan ensures that you know what to eat and how much to consume. The Pegan diet is straightforward because the restrictions are markedly less rigid.

A proper Paleo diet may be too difficult and expensive for some individuals. Considering the health implications, it is also a cause for concern. Veganism, on the other hand, is similarly strict and challenging to adhere to. As a result of combining these two contradictory diets, the Pegan diet, which provides a great balance of health benefits and minimal restrictions, makes a lot of sense for those of us who wish to live a healthy lifestyle while consuming a limited quantity of animal-based Protein.

The Pegan Diet incorporates the most beneficial characteristics of veganism and paleo nutrition. Gluten, dairy, soy, maize, potatoes, rice, and sugar are advised to be avoided. On the Pegan Diet, animal products are viewed as an occasional indulgence rather than a primary source of nutrition, promoting the consumption of more vegetables and fruits.

The majority of diets aid in weight loss by restricting calorie consumption and reducing hunger. The Pegan Diet permits complete appetite regulation by consuming more nutrient-dense foods, such as high-quality vegetables, and reducing total calories through natural caloric reduction or exercise. It has been demonstrated to have a significantly greater effect on satiety, allowing individuals to feel fuller for longer and resist appetites.

The Pegan Diet places an emphasis on flexibility. Pegans can adapt their diet to their lifestyle and vice versa, enabling them to enjoy food so long as it adheres to the 13 tenets of the Pegan Diet. It also means that if you dine out with a friend, you can still appreciate your meal knowing that the next day will be filled with fruits and vegetables.

Let's examine the thirteen pillars of the Pegan diet:

Sugar should be avoided at all costs. It entails avoiding sugar, wheat, and processed carbohydrates, all of which raise insulin levels. Sugar should be viewed as an occasional indulgence that should be consumed in moderation. It ought to be considered a recreational substance. It is something you do occasionally for fun, but it is not something you regularly imbibe. The majority of your diet consists of vegetation. As stated previously, vegetables should comprise more than half of one's tray. The denser the hue, the greater its intensity. The greater the variety, the better. Utilize vegetables with a high non-starch content. Winter squashes and sweet potatoes can be consumed in moderation (12 servings per day), but in excess should be avoided. Despite being the most popular vegetable in the United States, French fries do not qualify.

Fruit should not be consumed. It is the point of possible confusion. Vegan activists advocate consuming all fruit, whereas Paleo adherents advise consuming only low-sugar fruits such as cherries. The majority of Pegan followers appear to feel better when they adhere to low-glycemic foods and consider the rest a treat. Avoid consuming berries, kiwis, watermelon, grapes, melons, and other similar fruits. Consider desiccated fruit to be a sweet, and consume it sparingly.

Avoid using pesticides, antibiotics, hormones, and genetically modified organisms (GMOs). Prohibited substances include chemicals, preservatives, additives, pigments, artificial sweeteners, and potentially hazardous compounds. If an ingredient is absent from your kitchen, you should not consume it.

Consume foods high in wholesome fats. Nuts, legumes, olive oil, and avocados, to name a few, are rich sources of omega-3 fatty acids and other healthful fats. Yes, saturated fat is found in fish, whole eggs, grass-fed or sustainably raised livestock, grass-fed butter or ghee, organic virgin coconut oil and coconut butter.

Avoid the majority of vegetable, nut, and seed oils, such as canola, sunflower, maize, grapeseed, and particularly soybean oil, which accounts for approximately 10 percent of your daily caloric intake. Small quantities of expeller- or cold-pressed nut and seed oils, such as sesame, macadamia, and walnut, may be used as condiments or flavorings. Avocado oil is ideal for cooking at elevated temperatures.

Avoid dairy products or ingest them in moderation. The majority of individuals do not benefit from dairy. If you dislike it, you should avoid it, with the exception of yogurt, kefir, ghee, grass-fed butter, and cheese. Try sheep or goat milk instead of bovine milk. Additionally, select organic and grass-fed meats whenever possible.

Meat and animal products should be served as a condiment, or "Condi-meat," as opposed to the primary dish. Meat should be a secondary dish, while vegetables should be the main attraction. Each entrée should not exceed 4 to 6 ounces in size. Typically, prepare three or four vegetable side dishes at any given time.

Consume seafood that has been responsibly reared or harvested and is low in mercury. Sardines, herring, anchovies, and salmon captured in the wild contain low levels of mercury and toxins. Additionally, they should be collected or grown in an environmentally responsible manner.

Gluten should be completely avoided. Since "Franken wheat" is the most common source of gluten, you should seek out wheat varieties like einkorn. If you are not gluten-intolerant, you should only consume wheat on uncommon occasions. Harvard's Dr. Alessio Fasano, the world's preeminent expert on gluten, has conducted research demonstrating that gluten damages the stomach, even in those who are not gluten-intolerant and have no symptoms.

Consume gluten-free whole grains in moderation. They continue to increase blood sugar levels and can induce autoimmunity in certain individuals. Grains can increase blood glucose levels. Black rice, teff, buckwheat, quinoa, and amaranth are low-glycemic grains that should be ingested in small amounts (about a half cup per meal). A diet devoid of grains and legumes may be essential for treating and curing type 2 diabetes, autoimmune disease, and digestive issues. • Beans should be consumed infrequently if you are on the 10-Day Detox Diet or a diabetic ketogenic diet. Lentils are the most superior legume. Large and starchy beans ought to be avoided. There is an abundance of fiber, protein, and minerals in beans. However, they may induce digestive issues in some people and their lectins and phytates may inhibit mineral absorption. If you have diabetes, a high-bean diet may cause your blood sugar levels to rise. The consumption of up to 1 cup per day is acceptable.

Test your strategy to make it more customized. What works for one individual may not work for another. According to experts, everyone should eventually collaborate with a qualified nutritionist to further personalize their diet through testing.

1.4 The Pegan Food Pyramid

VEGETABLES, HERBS, AND SPICES WITHOUT STARCH: Unlimited, the base of the pyramid, consists of non-starchy, colorful vegetables, seasonings, and herbs. It is preferable if there are many hues.

According to Mark, the antioxidants found in blue and purple vegetables, anthocyanins, may help combat aging. Broccoli and artichokes are examples of amazing green vegetables. As he asserts, "Artichokes contain potent detoxifying substances as well as prebiotics, which serve to nourish all the healthy bacteria in your gut. "Gut microbes are crucial for your overall health."

Fat That Is Healthful: The physician suggests three to five servings. While many individuals attribute their health issues to fat, "healthy fat" does exist.

If you adhere to the Pegan diet, pasta is off-limits.Almost all diets are exclusive. According to the doctor, the Pegan food pyramid includes everything, with an emphasis on quality.

Up to a cup of lentils and 4 to 6 ounces of animal protein provide protein.

Mark believes that high-quality animal protein, such as grass-fed beef and dairy products, wild-caught seafood (or sustainably farmed if you must consume farmed fish), and pasture-raised meats, should be included in the Pegan diet.

"You need to know where your food comes from," says Rach.

According to the doctor, it is extremely difficult to obtain the high-quality, concentrated Protein and vitamins such as B12 found in lean meats and fish on a strict vegetarian diet.

Carbohydrate-rich vegetables and organic food: 1 cup of low-glycemic natural product to 1 cup of lackluster vegetables

Mark claims that organic foods have a low glycemic index, citing blueberries, raspberries, strawberries, and pomegranates as examples of organic foods with a low glycemic index.

Winter squash and yams are examples of unappetizing vegetables that contain cancer-preventing carotenoids and compounds.

Grains Gluten-Free: 1/2 to 1 CUP

According to the doctor, you may ingest grains, but you should seek out "excellent" grains that are low in starch, glycemic index, and gluten, such as quinoa and wild rice.

1.5 Sample Menu for 14 Days

These are the four points to remember:

Fill your platter with superstar vegetables

Consume 1-2 servings of nutritious Fat

The majority of meals should contain at least a condiment-sized portion of protein.

It is preferable to avoid inflammatory foods as much as possible (the majority of grains, foods that induce gas or constipation, processed and packaged foods).

Barley Breakfast Bowl

Preparation Time: 5 minutes
Cooking time: 15minutes
Servings: 4

Ingredients:

- 1.1/2 cups pearl barley
- 3.3/4 cups water
- Large pinch salt
- 1.1/2 cups dried cranberries
- 3 cups sweetened vanilla plant-based milk
- 2 tablespoons slivered almonds (optional)

Directions:

1. Put the barley, water, and salt. Bring to a boil.

2. Divide the barley into 6 jars or single-serving storage containers. Attached the 1/4 cup of dried cranberries to each. Pour 1/2 cup of plant-based milk into each. Attached the 1 teaspoon of slivered almonds (if using) to each. Close the jars tightly with lids.

Pegan Diet Basics

Pegan Diet Basics is a in a cookbook that provides an overview of the Pegan Diet and how to adhere to its principles. The Pegan Diet emphasizes the consumption of whole, plant-based foods while permitting the consumption of some animal products. On the Pegan Diet, you should consume a variety of fruits, vegetables, nuts, seeds, and healthy fats, while avoiding processed foods, grains and legumes, added sugars, dairy, and vegetable oils. By incorporating these principles into your lifestyle and adhering to the Pegan Diet, you can improve your overall health, promote sustainable weight loss, and increase your vitality.

What to Consume on the Vegan Diet

The Pegan Diet is based on the consumption of whole, unadulterated, nutrient-dense, and toxin-free foods. Here are some examples of the sorts of foods you should strive to consume while following the Pegan Diet:

Fruits: Fruits are essential to the Pegan Diet due to their high vitamin, mineral, and antioxidant content. On the Pegan Diet, acceptable fruits include cherries, apples, pears, oranges, and melons.

Vegetables: Vegetables should be a staple of the Pegan Diet due to their high nutrient content and low calorie content. On the Pegan Diet, you can consume vegetables such as verdant greens, broccoli, cauliflower, sweet potatoes, and bell peppers.

Nuts and Seeds: Nuts and seeds are an excellent source of healthy fats and protein, making them a fantastic option for a Pegan Diet snack. On the Pegan Diet, acceptable nuts and seeds include almonds, hazelnuts, chia seeds, and pumpkin seeds.

Healthy Fats: Healthy fats are an essential component of the Pegan Diet, as they provide energy and aid in nutrient absorption. On the Pegan Diet, some examples of healthful fats include avocado, olive oil, coconut oil, and ghee.

High-Quality Animal Products While the Pegan Diet is predominantly plant-based, it does permit the consumption of certain high-quality animal products. Regarding animal products, it is essential to prioritize quality over quantity.

Avoidable foods on the Pegan Diet

On the Pegan Diet, certain substances should be avoided in order to promote optimal health and support long-term weight loss. These consist of:

Processed foods are high in additives and preservatives and can be difficult to digest. They are prohibited on the Pegan Diet.

Grains and Legumes: While grains and legumes can be consumed in moderation as part of a nutritious diet, they should be limited on the Pegan Diet. This is due to the fact that they can be inflammatory and inhibit digestion.

Added Sugars: Many processed foods contain added sugars, which can contribute to a variety of health problems. They are prohibited on the Pegan Diet.

Dairy Products: Dairy products are typically excluded from the Pegan Diet due to the fact that they can be challenging to digest and contribute to inflammation.

Vegetable Oils: Soybean oil, corn oil, and canola oil are rich in omega-6 fatty acids, which may contribute to inflammation. These oils are prohibited on the Pegan Diet.

By avoiding these substances on the Pegan Diet, you can promote optimal health and long-term weight loss. Focus on whole, unprocessed foods, such as fruits, vegetables, nuts, seeds, and healthful fats, that are high in nutrients and low in toxins.

Meal Preparation and Planning for the Vegan Diet

Meal planning and preparation are essential for success on the Pegan Diet, as they help to ensure that you receive all of the necessary nutrients and have healthful options available when you're pressed for time. One of the most effective methods for planning and preparing meals on the Pegan Diet is to plan your meals and snacks in advance and compile an inventory of the necessary ingredients. This will assist you in staying on track and avoiding unhealthy food choices.

Another effective strategy is to cook a little excess food and store the leftovers for later use. This can save you time and money, as well as guarantee that you always have a wholesome option available when you are pressed for time. A slow cooker is an excellent tool for meal preparation on the Pegan Diet because it enables you to forget about it. Simply toss in an assortment of whole, unprocessed ingredients and let the slow cooker do the work while you attend to other matters.

Lastly, it is essential to stock your kitchen with an assortment of whole, nutrient-dense foods, including fruits, vegetables, nuts, seeds, and healthy lipids. This will make it simpler to adhere to the Pegan Diet, as healthy options will always be available. By adhering to these tips, you can effectively plan and prepare meals on the Pegan Diet and reap all of the health benefits that this unique diet has to offer.

The fundamentals of the vegan diet

Are you certain you're prepared to begin the vegan diet?You may have informed your family members (domestic members) about your new diet in order to prepare them for this carb-reduction diet. Let me not trouble you with the headache, irritability, uncontrollable fatigue, and cravings that frequently accompany the elimination of carbohydrates from the diet. You could attempt creating a meal plan for a couple of days, along with a grocery list tailored to the recipes you will need.

Healthiest diet

For those who are curious as to why the pegan diet is gaining popularity, it may be of interest to know that it is one of the healthiest scientifically proved effective diets.

Recent research suggests that the first five healthiest foods include the following: the Low-carb, whole-food diet, which is promoted primarily for people who want to lose weight and reduce the risk of disease infection for optimal health; the Mediterranean diet, the Paleo diet, the Vegan diet, and the Gluten-free diet.

Foods permitted on the Pegan Diet

As you will soon discover, the pegan diet strongly promotes whole foods or foods that undergo minimal or no processing before consumption. As you may have surmised, this is why plants appear to play a larger role in the pegan diet.

Vegetables and fruits should account for 75% of your total caloric intake throughout the period, as they are recommended to be your primary source of nutrition.

Fruits and vegetables with a low glycemic index, such as non-starchy vegetables, berries, and the like, are encouraged to reduce a single blood sugar response.

People who have attained healthy blood sugar regulation prior to beginning the diet are often permitted to consume a small amount of starchy vegetables and sweet fruits.

As stated previously, the healthy protein source should make up the majority of the remaining 25% of your diet after fruits and vegetables account for 75%.

Again, you are expected to maintain minimally processed lipids, also known as healthy fats from sources such as:

The Nuts besides peanuts

Excluding refined seed oils, the Seeds

Avocados and olives, including olive and avocado cold-pressed oils

Coconut-unrefined coconut oil is permitted as well.

Omega-3 fatty acids, with an emphasis on low-mercury fish or algae

In addition to pasture-raised meats and whole eggs, you may also consider pasture-raised meats and eggs for the lipid content of your vegan diet.

You may consume certain whole grains and legumes, particularly gluten-free whole grains and legumes, but only in very small amounts; the majority of these foods are prohibited due to their effect on blood sugar.

It is estimated that grain intake should not exceed 1/2 cup or 125 grams per meal, just as legume intake should not exceed 1 cup or 75 grams per meal.

Among the few grains and legumes you might contemplate consuming are:

For cereals, we recommend black rice, millet, quinoa, teff, oats, and amaranth.

For legumes, there are black beans, lentils, pinto beans, and chickpeas.

Patients with diabetes or other medical conditions that promote poor blood sugar regulation should avoid grains and legumes.

Bottom of the Form Pegan Diet, Avoid These Foods

Those who wish to follow the pegan diet should comprehend its tenets and be aware of the foods that are prohibited or, at the very least, discouraged due to their nutritional value or relative effect on the body.

Things like:

Sugar Gluten Dairy

Canola, soy, corn, or grapeseed oil.

Anything that has been exposed to pesticides, hormones, dyes, genetically modified organisms, artificial sweeteners, antibiotics, or preservatives should not be consumed.

As a Rule of Thumb for this Diet, you should always do the following:

Reduce starchy vegetables, such as potatoes and winter squash, to less than a half-cup per day while ingesting only low-sugar fruits, such as berries and kiwis. If you must consume legumes, you should consume less than a cup per day.

Whole grains that do not contain gluttons, such as teff, black rice, quinoa, and amaranth, should also be consumed with caution, no more than one-half cup per meal.

You may occasionally consume honey or sugar in the form of maple syrup.

You can also occasionally consume grass-fed, organic dairy products such as ghee and kefir. When there are no reports of discomfort-related side effects, sheep and goat milk products may also be consumed.

Every substance consumed should be minimally processed, with the majority of its natural constituents still intact.

Although the pegan diet does not specifically prohibit alcohol, the paleo diet does.

Are you perplexed by the selection of vegan foods?

Well, many adherents of the Pegan Diet claim they would have to literally read every label when purchasing in order to identify, for example, whole, organic, or sugar-free products.

Even more perplexing is determining which of the numerous options are minimally processed foods, not to mention understanding what the term addictive has to do with their selection, and then answering these and numerous other questions. Dr. Williams concludes, "There is no actual definition of 'clean' or 'processed,'... Even if you purchase cow's milk or raw poultry breasts, there is processing involved. Technically, even extra-virgin olive oil is refined. I attempt to steer people toward minimally processed, as close to their natural state as possible foods. When I examine the ingredient list, I ask myself: If I were to make this at home, would these ingredients be included? I'm searching for chemicals, colorings, and added carbohydrates, as well as other industrialized chemicals that aren't necessarily required for the food's production. They do not contribute to the nutritional value or stability of the product."

You desire to know how it tastes? Why not attempt the 14-day diet described in detail?

Disadvantages

Although the pegan diet has positive benefits, there are also some drawbacks to consider.

Undue restrictions

Although a pegan diet is more flexible than a vegan or paleo diet alone, it restricts healthful foods like legumes, whole grains, and dairy.

Increased inflammation and elevated blood sugar are frequently cited by proponents of pegan diets as the primary reasons for eliminating these foods.

Obviously, some individuals are allergic to gluten and dairy, which can cause inflammation. Similarly, some individuals have difficulty regulating their blood sugar after consuming foods with a high starch content, such as grains or legumes.

In such cases, it may be prudent to reduce or eliminate consumption of these substances. However, there is no need to avoid them unless you have specific food allergies or intolerances.

In addition, the random elimination of large food groups can result in nutrient deficiencies if these nutrients are not meticulously replaced. Therefore, a fundamental understanding of nutrition may be required to implement a pegan diet safely.

7 days Sample menu on pegan diet

Vegetables are encouraged on the pegan diet, which also includes meat, fish, legumes, and seeds. A moderate amount of gluten-free cereals and legumes may be consumed.

This is an example of a weekday menu:

Monday

Vegetable omelet with olive oil salad for breakfast

Kale salad with chickpeas, strawberries, and avocado for lunch.

Dinner of wild salmon with vegetables Roasted carrots, steamed broccoli, and balsamic vinegar made with citrus

Sweet potato "Tostada" with sliced avocado, pumpkin seeds, and lemon balsamic vinegar for breakfast on Tuesday.

Bento box containing boiled eggs, sliced turkey, raw vegetable segments, fermented kimchi, and Blackberries for lunch.

Dinner: cashews, shallots, bell peppers, tomatoes, and black beans stir-fried with vegetables

Wednesday

Green smoothie with pears, kale, almond butter, and hemp seeds for breakfast.

Lunch: Vegetable stir-fried remnants

Dinner: Grilled seafood and vegetable skewers Accompanied by black rice pilaf

Coconut and chia seed pudding with hazelnuts and fresh blueberries for breakfast on Thursday.

Mixed vegetable salad with avocado, cucumber, roasted chicken, and apple cider vinegar tea for lunch.

Salad of roasted beets, pumpkin seeds, Brussels sprouts, and sliced almonds for supper.

Friday's breakfast consists of scrambled eggs, kimchi, and braised vegetables.

Lunch: lentils and vegetables stewed with diced cantaloupe

Grass-fed radish, jicama, guacamole, and julienne salad for dinner.

Overnight oatmeal with cashew milk, chia seeds, almonds, and berries for Saturday's breakfast.

The midday meal and remains lentil stewed vegetables

Pork loin roast served with steamed vegetables, vegetables, and quinoa

Sunday Breakfast: vegetable omelette and uncomplicated Green Salad

Thai Salad Roll with Cashew Cream Sauce and Orange Slice for Lunch

Dinner: Leftover Pork Tenderloin and Vegetables

Cool Tomato And Cucumber Gazpacho

(Prepping time: 10 minutes \ Cooking time: No-Cook Time |For 4 servings

Ingredients

- **8 ripe plum/heirloom tomatoes**
- **1 medium red bell pepper, seeded and coarsely chopped**
- **1 medium cucumber, coarsely chopped**
- **½ cup extra virgin olive oil**
- **1 tablespoon balsamic/red wine vinegar**
- **Salt and pepper as needed**
- **Sunflower seeds for garnish**

Directions

1. Take your food processor and add tomatoes, pepper, cucumber, and pulse until everything breaks down

2. While the motor is still running, add oil, the process for about 2 minutes until the mix is smooth and velvety

3. Add vinegar and process for a few seconds more

4. Refrigerate the soup for about 2 hours, serve cold with a bit of salt and pepper

5. Garnish with some seeds if desired

6. Enjoy!

Pegan Det A Healthu Selection For You?

Since a regular diet does not specify how much you can eat in a given day, it does not necessarily comply with the USDA's guidelines for daily calories, macronutrients, and micronutrients. You should be able to meet these needs while adhering to the diet's list of permitted ingredients with careful planning.

If you're trying to lose weight, knowing your daily calorie needs will help you stay on track with your objectives.

Health Advantages

Dr. Human suggests that the health benefits of plant-based and raleo diets are comparable. In fact, research indicates that a plant-based diet can aid in the treatment and prevention of several types of cancer, as well as promote weight loss.7 In addition, raleo diets are associated with weight loss and the management of Parkinson's disease, but more research is required to ascertain their long-term health effects.

However, there is no evidence that combining these two diets and restricting certain food groups will produce superior health outcomes than a balanced diet. A 2016 study of a large sample revealed that dairy fat was not associated with the risk of sardovasular deae, despite the fact that dairy fat is sometimes criticized for its high saturated fat content.

The Health Rk

Although there are no known health risks associated with a paleo diet because it is still a relatively new eating pattern, eliminating dairy and whole cereals may result in nutrient deficiencies. Cow's milk contains significant amounts of sodium, protein, potassium, and vitamin D, all of which are essential for good health.

In addition, whole grains are an excellent source of fiber, vitamins, and minerals. A 2016 landmark study found that consuming whole grains reduces the risk of heart disease, cancer, and all-cause mortality.10 Additional studies have demonstrated that a deficiency in thiamine, folate, magnesium, sodium, iron, and iodine can result from a diet deficient in these foods.

Beans provide numerous benefits and are widely regarded as a healthy diet due to their fiber, protein, and phytonutrient content.12 Beans are an excellent source of plant-based protein for vegan diets. The elimination of legumes from a diet puts 75% of trend-based diet followers at risk for insufficient protein, fiber, and other essential nutrients.

How Should I Proceed?

There are specific rules and regulations associated with the regan diet, and adhering to them is essential.

Eat Tons Of Vegetables

Vegetables and fruits should make up more than half of each meal, as the purpose of the vegan diet is to cleanse the body and introduce healthy nutrients.

Clean diet will not only help you maintain a healthy body, but it will also revitalize your skin. Truly incorporating seasonal fruits and vegetables into your diet. Variety of produce will keer your interest intake.

Choose Animal Proten

Foods to enhanse uour beauty

Your meal should contain an adequate amount of high-quality animal protein. These protein-rich foods include eggs, beef, lean meat, olive oil, etc. Since they come with their own benefits, eliminating them will deprive your body of protein-rich foods.

Be Patient

Pegan det refers to the long journey. You will not see many results in a shorter period of time. Your body will need time to adjust to the new regimen and produce the desired results. Therefore, be patient, continue your good effort, and do not lose hope. It will be harsh.

Choose Prorortional Wages

The rrororton rlau plays an essential role here. Before embarking on a raw food diet, you should consult with a nutritionist to determine whether or not a raw food diet and regimen are suitable for your body.

Say No To Drug Users

Tips for a healthy summer diet

Gluten should not be on your menu if you choose to follow a vegetarian diet. Gluten-based foods increase the amount of fat in the body and cause you to gain excessive amounts of weight. Therefore, avoiding whole-grain breads, cereals, rice, and brown rice will benefit your health even more.

Prepare Your Meal Yourself

It will help you understand your body better if you prepare your meals on your own. In addition, cooking for yourself will reassure you that you've been consuming a healthy diet because everything will be in front of your eyes.

One more reason to cook at home will help you save a ton of money, as the food items required for a conventional diet are prohibitively expensive. There are numerous recipes for regan det available on the Internet. Theu are simple, delisious and somrletelu in uour budget.

Cravings

Theu may take a toll on you at times, but you should resist giving in to your desires and steadfastly adhere to the plan.

Replacing certain food items with their healthier alternatives can address many of your problems, such as switching from cow's milk to goat's milk, which is easier to digest, or choosing coconut yogurt or vegan cheese.

Strawberry Balsamic Chicken and Spinach Salad
Servings: 4

Ingredients:
- 6 to 8 cups chopped baby spinach
- 1 ¾ cups sliced strawberries
- 2 grilled chicken breast halves, sliced thin (optional)
- 3 tablespoons olive oil
- 2 tablespoons balsamic vinegar
- Pinch dry mustard powder
- Pinch salt

Instructions:
1. Divide the spinach among four salad plates.
2. Sprinkle all but ¼ cup of the strawberries over the salads as evenly as possible.
3. Divide the sliced chicken among the salads – skip this step if you are not using chicken.
4. Combine the remaining ingredients in a food processor.

5.   Blend the mixture until smooth then drizzle over the salads to serve.

Differences Between Paleo, Pegan And Vegan Diet

The pegan diet incorporates the vegan and paleo eating styles. The vegan diet's stringent commitment to animal-free eating and the paleo diet's reputation for a meat-centric diet appear to be diametrically opposed. The pegan diet seeks to combine the best of both worlds despite this. Is it feasible, and how does it function? Let's examine more closely.

The pegan diet adopts the plant-based philosophy of the vegan diet and the meat-centric philosophy of the caveman-inspired paleo diet. If you're unfamiliar with the paleo diet, it attempts to replicate what Paleolithic humans ate 2.6 million years ago: vegetables, fruits, fish, meat, and nuts. Not permitted are dairy, wheat, legumes, sugar, oils, salt, alcohol, and caffeine. Veganism, on the other hand, prohibits the consumption of animal-based foods and mandates the consumption of only plant-based foods. The fundamental principle of the vegan diet is to emphasize whole foods while excluding refined foods. Particularly, the pegan diet requires that 75 percent of calories come from plant sources, with the remaining 25 percent originating from animal sources.

Is there anything else I ought to know?

Yes, indeed. While the pegan diet's emphasis on plant-based foods is beneficial, other of its stringent guidelines have not been shown to be healthy. Gluten, for instance, is prohibited on this diet despite the absence of a valid medical condition such as celiac disease or gluten sensitivity. Gluten is restricted for various nonscientific reasons. During the Paleolithic period, for instance, milling technology was not yet developed, so cereals were not consumed by cavemen. It is also avoided for reasons that have not yet been demonstrated in the diet literature. Gluten-free grains such as quinoa, brown rice, oats, and amaranth may be ingested, but in moderation and in limited quantities.

On the vegan diet, dairy products are prohibited and legumes are severely restricted. This diet also encourages the consumption of grass-fed, pasture-raised animal products and the purchase of organic produce and other items. As many additives, chemicals, preservatives, artificial colors, flavors, and sweeteners as possible should be avoided by Pegan adherents. By minimizing these elements, the pegan diet emphasizes "clean" eating, a trendy buzzword for a way of eating with no concrete meaning and therefore no research-documented impact on health.

Pegan Diet

A pegan diet is essentially a combination of the paleo and vegan regimens.

A vegan diet excludes all animal products and their derivatives, such as meat, milk, cheese, yogurt, and gelatin. A paleo diet is a diet based on what humans ate during the Paleolithic period, 2.5 million years ago. Dieters consume more whole foods, such as vegetables, fruits, nuts, grass-fed meats, and salmon.

What distinguishes the pegan diet from the vegan and ketogenic diets?

While vegan and paleo diets appear to be at odds with one another – one promotes avoiding dairy, meat, and fish, while the other promotes eating meat and fish – the foundation of both lifestyles is the consumption of whole foods and vegetation.

The purpose of the pegan diet is to promote individuals to consume more fresh, organic, and whole foods, as well as to increase their vegetable consumption.

The pegan diet also emphasizes the quality of the foods you consume, promoting individuals to consume organic foods.

What are your eating plans?

Plants, specifically.

Nuts and seeds, healthy fats, and vegetables can make up the preponderance of your diet.

The doctor clarified that 75% of the diet should consist of fruits and vegetables, while dairy and gluten should be avoided.

If you must consume dairy, the diet suggests ewe or goat milk products.

What are the benefits?

Although the pegan diet is not for everyone, it has been shown to assist certain individuals.

Marlowe stated, "I grew up eating a typical American diet, which led to a multitude of health problems." "Eating pegan helped me lose 20 pounds, eliminate digestive problems, increase my stamina, and improve my overall health."

Vegan Diet

A vegan diet consists of plants (such as vegetables, grains, nuts, and fruits) and plant-based goods.

Vegans abstain from plant-based foods, such as dairy and eggs.

As a vegan, you should consume healthy foods.

A varied and healthful vegan diet can provide the majority of essential nutrients.

For a vegan diet that is both healthy and tasty:

At least five portions of a variety of fruits and vegetables should be consumed daily.

Potatoes, bread, rice, pasta, and other starchy carbohydrates may be used as meal foundations (when practicable, opt for whole grains).

There are dairy substitutes available, such as soy milk and yogurt (choose those with less cholesterol and sugar).

Consume a portion of legumes and other protein-rich dishes.

Choose oils and condiments that are unsaturated and consume in moderation.

The government recommends 6 to 8 cups or pints of water per day.

If you choose to consume foods and beverages that are high in fat, sodium, or sugar, do so in moderation.

Vegan calcium and vitamin D sources

Calcium is essential for healthy bones and teeth.

Non-vegans obtain the majority of their calcium from dairy products (milk, cheese, and yogurt), but vegans can obtain calcium from a variety of sources.

For vegans, calcium-rich foods include spinach fortified soy, rice, and oat beverages. Green, leafy vegetables — such as broccoli, cabbage, and okra, but not spinach — fortified soya, rice, and oat beverages that are not sweetened.

Tofu calcium-set sesame seeds and tahini bread (both brown and white) (in the United Kingdom, calcium is required to be added to white and brown flour).

Dried fruit includes raisins, prunes, figs, and dried apricots, among others.

A 30g portion of dried fruit counts as one of your five daily servings, but it should be consumed at mealtimes rather than as a snack between meals to minimize the impact of sugar on teeth.

The body requires vitamin D to regulate calcium and phosphate levels. These nutrients aid in the maintenance of healthy bones, teeth, and tendons.

Vitamin D can be obtained from the following vegan-friendly sources:

Exposition to sunlight, especially from late March/early April to the end of September – Remember to cover or shield your skin before it turns crimson or burns (see vitamin D and sunlight).

Vitamin D is added to unsweetened soy beverages, fortified fat condiments, and breakfast cereals.

dietary supplementation with vitamin D

Verify on the label that the vitamin D in a food is not derived from animals.

sources of iron for vegans

Iron is required for red blood cell formation.

Even though the body absorbs iron from plant-based foods less efficiently than iron from livestock, a vegan diet may be high in iron.

Iron-rich vegan foods consist of dark green, verdant vegetables like watercress, broccoli, and spring greens. Dried fruits include apricots, prunes, and figs Apricots, prunes, and figs are examples of wholemeal bread and flour breakfast cereals fortified with iron.

Vitamin B12 plant-based sources

The body requires vitamin B12 to maintain healthy circulation and a healthy nervous system.

Vitamin B12 is typically derived from animal products like poultry, fish, and dairy. Due to a dearth of available sources, vegans may require a vitamin B12 supplement.

The following foods provide vegans with vitamin B12:

Vitamin B12 yeast extract fortified soy beverages, such as Marmite, which is fortified with vitamin B12. sources of omega-3 fatty acids that are vegan

Omega-3 fatty acids, such as those found in oily fish, can help maintain a healthy heart and reduce the risk of heart disease when consumed as part of a balanced diet.

Omega-3 fatty acids are available to vegans from the following sources:

Oil extracted from flaxseed (Linseed).

Rapeseed Oil

Soybean Oil and Soy-Based Foods, Such as Tofu

According to research, plant sources of omega-3 fatty acids do not have the same benefits in reducing the risk of heart disease as those found in oily fish.

Vegans can take care of their hearts by eating at least five servings of a variety of fruits and vegetables daily, avoiding foods high in saturated fat, and monitoring their sodium intake.

Benefits Of A Pegan Diet

This diet's primary objective is to combine the nutrients found in animal products, such as omega 3, vitamin B12, lipids, protein, and iron, with those found in plant products, such as vitamins, minerals, fiber, and phytochemicals. A pegan diet fully satisfies protein requirements because it includes plant sources such as legumes (which have more protein than grains) and replaces some of the animal food groups with plant-based foods, allowing people who would not be able to follow a Paleo or Vegan diet to do so without suffering from food deprivation. The Pegan diet is an all-inclusive eating plan!

Elimination of manufactured goods

The main advantage of a vegan diet is its ability to exclude processed foods, which not only provide our bodies with few nutrients but also, due to their high sugar content and artificial ingredients such as dyes, refined sugars, salts, artificial flavors, preservatives, and flavor enhancers, are the main cause of our psychophysical imbalance and the leading cause of cardiovascular diseases, cancers, diabetes, obesity, and diseases of the endocrine system. The vast majority of these products, including cereals, snacks, pasta sauces, frozen meals, salad dressings, crackers, ice cream, and cake mixtures, contain artificial food coloring, and the majority of packaged and industrial foods have a high glycemic index and a low satiety index. This means that they are not satisfying in terms of satisfaction and satiety, but rather temporarily fill the stomach without providing nutrients to our bodies; after a brief time, hunger returns, and we are forced to reopen the refrigerator in search of food. Processed foods respond to the profit motive of large multinational corporations that strive for a standard and industrial food supply, as fresh and perishable foods translate to less profit for them due to their short shelf life and poor portability.

A sustainable diet

The km 0 aspect

In order to avoid consuming foods containing chemicals, additives, and pesticides, one of the cardinal principles of the Pegan diet is to prioritize the consumption of local and 0-kilometer foods, products of certified and organic origin, and seasonal foods. Therefore, local food whose producer guarantees its authenticity is preferable over global products that frequently lack origin certification. This model contributes to the reevaluation of land, its rediscovery, and the conservation of natural resources. The preference for local products is a response to the globalization of food production, which has diminished the quality and availability of local food. In addition to providing consumers with more sustainable, healthier, and fresher food options, the pro-local km 0 movement generates economic benefits for small farmers and businesses and enhances cooperation and support among local producers. Trading local produce is not just about consuming food produced in the same geographic region as the market where it is sold; it is also about supporting the people who produce it by purchasing their goods and learning about their histories and cultures.

In the Pegan diet, foods of animal origin are permitted so long as they originate from extensive farming, i.e., free-range and pasture-based, and were not raised on industrial feed but on grass and hay, referred to as Grass Fed products.

Another factor to consider when discussing km 0 is the decreased use of plastic packaging for transporting food, which contributes to the reduction of waste. In addition, with short-chain transportation, the costs and consumption associated with wrapping, washing, and packaging the food are amortized, and avoiding lengthy journeys reduces cold storage fuel and energy consumption. In conclusion, bringing food that is representative of one's region to the table is a conscious decision that considers sustainability and has long-lasting positive effects on the environment and on our health.

The seasonality of goods

By purchasing short-chain or 0-km products, we have the opportunity to consume wholesome and fresh foods that do not contain additional preservatives, as they have not been subjected to lengthy intercontinental journeys or sudden temperature and climate changes. The purchase of such items is closely tied to their seasonality: eating food in accordance with the season in which it ripens maximizes its nutritional value, as it contains the maximum concentration of vitamins and minerals during harvest. In addition, eating seasonally means respecting the natural cycle of nature and adapting to what the earth provides season by season, as our Paleolithic progenitors did, without the intervention of unsustainable agriculture. Due to greenhouses and intercontinental transportation, there is never a paucity of any type of produce, even when it is out of season, in large supermarket chains. Consequently, we are more likely to purchase the same vegetables or foods throughout the year. Out of season foods consist of those that ripen early or late, are cultivated in greenhouses with artificial light, are harvested while still unripe, and are treated with gas to prevent ripening. In addition to having a significant impact on the environment due to the extensive use of chemicals to speed up their growth, these foods also have a significant impact on our bodies. They are nutrient-depleted, water-filled foods with little flavor, and once digested, our bodies convert them into nitrates, which are extremely dangerous for the body because they reduce the amount of oxygen in the blood by affecting hemoglobin. Otherwise, by respecting seasonality, we will be "forced" to eat what nature provides in season, and we will be able to enjoy a wider variety of fruits and vegetables throughout the year. We will also be able to include in our diet a very rich range of fiber, antioxidants, phytonutrients, and vitamins, which help us to face the season in the best way and boost our immune system. The foods will have an unmistakable flavor and aroma due to their natural maturation without the use of artificial lighting. In the summer, for instance, we require more hydration, and nature provides us with watermelons, melons, peaches, and plums, which hydrate us, provide the proper amount of mineral salts, and aid our digestive system due to their fiber content. In the winter, vitamin C-rich citrus fruits, kiwis, citrons, cauliflower, and cabbage are needed to strengthen the immune system against severe weather and influenza.

Food as treatment

Foods can legitimately be regarded to have medicinal properties in numerous ways, including not only the prevention or treatment of disease, but also the promotion of health. The link between food and health is unavoidable, as humans have used food as a natural cure for disease and to preserve mental and physical health for centuries. The food we consume is the primary source of energy, strength, vigor, and vitality; food provides us with the resources necessary to live a healthful lifestyle.

According to Dr. Hyman, the pegana diet promotes healthy and sustainable weight loss, improves cholesterol levels, regulates blood sugar levels, and decreases the risk of diabetes, cardiovascular disease, and digestive diseases. As previously stated, through plants we can assimilate a large number of phytochemicals, a group of approximately 25,000 chemical compounds produced by plants as pest and pathogen defense. Recent studies demonstrate that phytochemicals are essential for humans as well, as they strengthen the immune system, reduce inflammation, and reduce the risk of developing cancer.

Dietary use of hues

A crucial aspect of the Pegan diet is consuming foods of various hues, as each color corresponds to a unique source of nutrients and beneficial properties for the body. It is necessary to consume fruits and vegetables from each color group every day. Each color category corresponds to distinct health benefits.

Fruits and vegetables are divided into five fundamental color categories:

Red: foods rich in vitamin C, carotenoids, anthocyanins, and lycopene, antioxidant-rich compounds. Anthocyanins, which promote blood circulation, are helpful in the fight against free radicals and in lowering harmful cholesterol levels. Recent research indicates that lycopene can prevent prostate cancer, cardiovascular disorders, breast cancer, and uterine cancer.

Yellow-orange: foods rich in beta-carotene, bioflavonoids, and vitamin C, which are precursors to vitamin A. By promoting healthy tissue, development, vision, and collagen formation, they have antioxidant and anti-aging effects on the epidermis. They also support metabolic processes.

Anthoxanthin-, polyphenol-, sulfur-, quercetin-, and flavonoid-rich foods are white. They aid in lowering levels of "bad" cholesterol and blood pressure, have antioxidant properties, and aid in waste elimination.

Chlorophyll, an antioxidant and anti-anemic substance, is abundant in green foods. They possess antianemic properties, promote calcium absorption, and combat aging. Rich in mineral ions, they stimulate the production of folic acid, vitamin C, and carotenoids, thereby promoting cell regeneration, bone health, dental health, and blood vessel health.

Blue-violet: foods abundant in anthocyanins, carotenoids, and resveratol, antioxidants that are beneficial for circulation and have anti-aging, diuretic, and purifying properties. They guard against cardiovascular disease, stroke, intestinal flora, and urinary tract infections.

To maximize the benefits of the color diet, you must pay close attention to the preparation methods of foods. It is best to consume them raw or in the form of extracts (cold extraction), but you can also choose non-invasive cooking methods such as steaming, low-temperature cooking, or quick pan searing. Avoid violent or prolonged preparation of vegetables; during boiling in water, the majority of organoleptic properties are lost in the cooking liquid, along with the majority of the benefits and nutrients.

Other advantages of the Pegan diet's foods include:

Weight reduction

Due to the low caloric content of the majority of plant foods, they can be consumed in large quantities to satiate hunger, and the fiber content will allow you to feel full for longer without consuming an excessive number of calories. Weight loss does not have to be the objective of the journey, but it will be a direct result of a diet that seeks to improve an individual's internal state of health by adopting a diet like Pegan's and leading a healthy lifestyle. If you maintain consistency, the results will be sustained over time. The secret to the Pegan diet is allowing the consumption of a variety of foods without deprivation but in moderation, so that you can begin it without experiencing the burden of a drastic and overly restrictive change. Psychological stress is a major contributor to weight gain, not weight loss; a state of psychophysical imbalance caused by forced overtraining, an iron-rich diet, and the resulting emotional stress does not aid weight loss. People tend to overeat and binge during periods of high stress; chronic stress also increases the risk of obesity. Eating under the influence of constant guilt, being in a state of emotional disarray, and being exhausted by the thought of having to lose weight at all costs stimulates the production of cortisol, the well-known "stress hormone," which raises blood sugar levels, causes abdominal bloating, and promotes the accumulation of fatty tissue, as well as making you feel even more exhausted mentally and physically.

Detoxification and antioxidant diet

According to the mitochondria theory, free radical oxidation causes cellular senescence. Mitochondria are the "power plants" of the cell, converting glucose and oxygen into usable energy for the remainder of the cell. Endosymbiosis is the process by which some cells obtain mitochondria from other cells, while others produce their own mitochondria. Antioxidants are substances that protect the cell by counteracting the infamous molecules known as free radicals; these antioxidants can be produced through a variety of means, including exercise and the consumption of natural antioxidants found in fruits and vegetables, such as vitamins A, C, E, selenium, carotenoids, lycopene, coenzyme Q-10, and lipoic acid. On average, plant-based foods contain 64 times as many antioxidants as animal-based foods. In light of this, the Pegan diet, which consists of 75 percent plant-based foods such as fruits, vegetables, herbs, and seasonings, allows you to experience a detoxifying and antioxidant effect throughout the entire day, every day. In addition, a low-calorie diet, such as the Pegan diet, can help you live longer and delay the aging of your cells: low-calorie diets reduce the amount of energy and oxygen that cells require, thereby reducing the number of free radicals produced by cells.

The Pegan diet has the unique characteristic of "cleansing" the body from the inside; meals based on fruits and vegetables aid in blood alkalinization and body detoxification. Fruit regulates blood sugar levels while protein and fiber stimulate digestion and prevent constipation.

Source of vitality and mental health

The high presence of fruits and vegetables in the pegana diet is a source of vitality, mental well-being, and happiness, and reduces the likelihood of developing mood-related symptoms. A diet rich in vitamins, minerals, and antioxidants can influence brain structure and function as well as mood, while at the same time protecting us from oxidative stress. Oxidative stress occurs when the free radicals produced by cellular reactions become excessive, causing damage to body cells and the brain. These nutrients contribute to a person's mental and physical health and emotional stability. Recent research indicates that excessive sugar consumption decreases serotonin levels in the brain, resulting in anxiety, melancholy, and low self-esteem.

Serotonin is a neurotransmitter that helps regulate sleep, temperament, appetite, and mood, and the majority of it is produced in the gut. The latter is lined with innumerable nerve cells, so it is logical to assume that the digestive system not only aids in the digestion of food but also in the regulation of emotions. Moreover, the functioning of digestive system cells and serotonin production are strongly influenced by the billions of "good" bacteria that form gut microbiome. So how can we keep the gut microbiome in shape?

The pegana diet is excellent for promoting the balance of our gut and preserving the "good" bacteria in the flora due to the presence of vegetables and fiber that promote intestinal motility thereby stimulating the production of neurotransmitters such as serotonin. Vegetables, fruits, legumes, olive oil and fish help to increase the presence of particular proteins that promote the development of new neurons in the hippocampus in the same way as antidepressant drugs but in a natural way. Omega-3s, on the other hand, help reduce the brain inflammation that often precedes the state of depression and mental malaise.

Health Benefits Of Eating Pegan

The pegan diet was developed with the objective of enhancing your health, well-being, and lifespan. By choosing nutrient-dense, whole foods over an excessively processed diet, you eliminate diseases, illnesses, and other health issues from your life immediately. Additionally, you enhance fat loss, vitality, and the production of feel-good chemicals. You will recommend this diet to everyone you meet due to the numerous significant health benefits associated with it.

Pegan to Lose Weight

Millions of individuals struggle with weight loss and wish to discover a solution. Thousands of fad diets promote 'immediate' and 'rapid' weight loss, but frequently leave dieters in a worse physical state than when they began. However, there is a solution to this terrible conflict that so many people face. The pegan diet will improve all aspects of your health, making weight loss effortless and straightforward.

Weight loss may be the first thing that comes to mind when you consider becoming healthier. Although the number on the scale is not the only indicator of health, being overweight can make it difficult for the body to perform essential functions. It places painful pressure on your joints, causes back pain, and increases your risk for hypertension, among many other illnesses.

It may appear challenging, if not impossible, to lose weight in order to achieve a healthful weight. Most people leave fad diets with damaged metabolisms and unsustainable habits, despite the fact that they promise quick and simple results. Studies indicate that the majority of lost weight is typically regained.

Adopting a vegan diet will serve as the wake-up call your body needs to start losing weight. By consuming a non-processed, plant-based diet with lean protein, you will discover that losing weight is actually quite simple. Let's discuss the science behind weight loss and how the pegan diet can help you achieve your weight loss goals.

The Science of Weight Management

Weight loss can appear to be an enigma. Without a true understanding of the mechanisms that regulate weight, reducing weight appears to be a mysterious and elusive process. Let's define weight loss and explain how the vegan diet can assist.

Calorie-wise, we lose weight when we consume fewer calories than we require. When you lose weight, your body loses substance. This mass is not always composed of fat, contrary to popular belief. Weight loss can also be comprised of muscle. This is why excess fat reduction is a superior objective to weight loss.

The metabolism plays a significant role in weight or fat loss. Metabolism refers to the series of cellular chemical reactions that convert sustenance into energy. The rate at which these reactions occur, or the rate at which you expend calories, is your metabolic rate. Some individuals have a naturally robust metabolism and can burn calories more quickly.

What exactly are calories? And is daily calorie monitoring essential? Calories are energy units. According to the official Merriam-Webster definition, a calorie is "the amount of heat required at a pressure of one atmosphere to raise the temperature of one gram of water by one degree Celsius" (2021). Simply put, a calorie is the amount of energy provided by sustenance. It is a measure of the energy impact of food on the human organism as a whole. Men require approximately 2,500 calories per day, while women require approximately 2,000.

How can the Pegan Diet assist me in weight loss?

Consuming fewer calories and exercising more will result in weight loss. Nonetheless, this has nothing to do with disease prevention, inflammation prevention, or increasing longevity. Certainly, burning more calories will result in weight loss. However, if you do not consume nutrient-dense foods, you may still experience inflammation, digestive issues, and be at risk for disease.

With the pegan diet, you can both lose weight and significantly improve your health. By consuming a plant-based diet, you consume foods that are naturally low in calories and have numerous other health benefits. For instance, consuming legumes also results in the consumption of Butyrate, which has been shown to reduce cancer risk and increase metabolic rate. various foods contain various chemical compounds with differing health benefits, but they all affect our body's ability to lose weight rapidly.

Our metabolism is slowed by the modern human diet, which consists primarily of processed foods. This can be observed at a microscopic level in the mitochondria of the cell. Mitochondria are cellular factories that generate energy. When food is digested, the molecular vitamins, nutrients, and minerals are fed to the mitochondria for energy production. This process requires a particular set of vitamins and nutrients, the majority of which are absent from processed, nutrient-poor diets.

Consequently, the energy output of each of our cells declines. We cannot have fast metabolisms to burn fat if we consume processed, nutrient-deficient foods. Therefore, it is essential to consume vegetables rich in B vitamins, zinc, and magnesium, among other nutrients. Eating broccoli, blackberries, and pomegranates will increase your metabolism and make it simpler to lose weight.

If you simply restricted calories, you would lose weight, but your body would eventually endure. This is the tragedy behind most novelty diets that drastically reduce calorie consumption. With such an abrupt decrease in energy intake, your metabolism recovers at a slower rate. In the beginning, a caloric deficit works well for the majority of people, but as the body attempts to prevent malnutrition and adjusts the metabolism, weight loss levels off.

In most countries, including the United States, fast food restaurants are ubiquitous. When creating recipes for their establishments, these corporations do not have your health in mind. They are intent on profit maximization. They want you to become addicted to their cuisine so that you return frequently and crave the same flavors. Fast-food restaurants use large quantities of salt, sugar, and added fats to trick the brain into desiring more.

This delicious food raises your insulin levels, increases your blood sugar, and triggers the release of "happy chemicals" in the brain. This immediate surge you get from biting into a greasy hamburger is even more irresistible when you're under pressure. The reason for this is that when we are agitated, our levels of happy chemicals such as dopamine are low. Fast food makes us temporarily feel better and compels us to consume when we are overworked, exhausted, or anxious.

When advertisements and fast food restaurants display appetizing-looking food everywhere, it is challenging to lose weight. Typically, the delicacies depicted in photographs are not even sustenance. They have been designed and edited to pique your interest. What you receive in the store will bear no resemblance to the image. Having to resist the temptation to stop at a fast-food restaurant hinders our efforts to lose weight. Moreover, many locations exist in a "food desert" where healthful food options and specific food categories are scarce. Instead, fast food restaurants and processed foods are the most accessible and practical options. This reality, which is overlooked by some, makes becoming healthier more difficult.

Many people believe that more pressure is placed on consumers to make healthful decisions when large corporations make it exceedingly difficult for them to do so. The cuisine they serve is more of a profit-maximizing scientific endeavor. When this is the goal, compounds are added to produce the intended flavor and appearance. However, the damage to your digestive system, metabolism, and overall health is irreversible.

Additionally, processed foods are ubiquitous in supermarkets. Sugar and dangerous additives that would not normally be present are present in these products. Labels such as "natural" are not regulated by the FDA, so consumers purchase them under the assumption that they are healthful. In actuality, declaring a product to be natural does not restrict the ingredients it may contain. 'Healthy' food is frequently a marketing term as opposed to a true claim. The use of muted earthy tones, minimal font, and terms like 'natural,' 'healthy,' and 'nature' deceive the consumer into believing they are making a good choice.

Therefore, consuming pegan is your best option. Avoid products with long lists of ingredients and undetermined side effects. Avoid the grocery store's processed food turmoil. By consuming unprocessed, whole foods, you can determine if they are safe to eat without reading the label.

Eating plant-based foods that are low in calories and high in essential nutrients is the most effective method to lose weight, increase metabolism, and prevent disease and health problems. These nutrients provide everything your body requires.

Diet Culture vs. Lifestyle Change

As a means of weight reduction, the pegan diet is not a quick fix. As stated previously, this is a new lifestyle change in which you prioritize consuming in a way that is beneficial to your body.

It can be difficult to distinguish between new diets in our society of frequent novelty diets and rapid weight loss solutions. If you are trying to lose weight, you may revert to an old strategy and yearn for a quick cure.

It is imperative to shift your focus from pursuing immediate results on the scale to how you feel. A number on the scale does not reveal an individual's health in its entirety. Due to their relentless pursuit of this number, numerous individuals have developed eating disorders and obsessions.

One strategy for resolving this issue is to abandon the scale entirely and pursue alternative methods for measuring success. This may include fitting into a smaller size of apparel or experiencing increased energy throughout the day. Changes such as enhanced facial skin and shinier hair may become apparent. It is crucial to acknowledge that success is not always quantifiable.

We have been conditioned to believe that weight is the most important factor in determining health by the diet culture. Despite the fact that it helps our bodies function, there are numerous other considerations to take into account. Diet culture makes losing weight more about looking good to impress others than improving one's quality of life.

A change in lifestyle, in contrast, focuses on you and your mental and physical health. If you want to feel energized, be happier, and live a longer, disease-free existence, you must immediately alter your diet. Consumption is converted into energy and mass. It is time to change your diet and significantly improve your quality of life.

Pegan Anti-Inflammatory

A reduction in inflammation is an additional extremely advantageous health benefit of adopting a vegan lifestyle. The body develops a variety of health problems in response to a typical diet of fast food, junk food, and excessively processed foods. Numerous aspects of our lives are affected by inflammation, including acne, bothersome joints, and digestive issues.

Inflammation is a widespread health issue that affects millions of individuals. By adopting a vegan diet, you can anticipate the elimination of these issues. Your skin, ligaments, and digestive system will become healthier. Your body will spend less time determining what to do with so many excess carbohydrates and artificial substances and more time helping you feel your best.

Internal inflammation of the human body

In light of all this talk about inflammation in the body, it is essential to define inflammation.

The immune system's response to numerous physiological events is inflammation. When exposed to a pathogen or an infection, the body's immune system is activated, resulting in inflammation. Inflammation also provides epidermis protection. When ultraviolet (UV) rays cause injury, blood cells heal the area, causing it to appear red and occasionally swollen. This demonstrates inflammation.

In an attempt to repel an invading virus or bacterium, your immune system will attack the cells in your digestive tract if your inflammatory system is out of whack. Inflammation of the gastrointestinal tract is a complex biological response to bacteria, damaged cells, or irritants that have caused injury. Many digestive issues, including Irritable Bowel Syndrome, may be brought on by excessive inflammation.

In numerous diseases, such as arthritis, the immune system is activated despite the absence of a threat. This causes joint and bone discomfort for no apparent reason. In other instances, such as inflammation resulting from digestion, the body breaks down food that it cannot metabolize. Constipation, irregularity, bloating, and diarrhea are some of the symptoms caused by inflammation.

However, you can resolve nearly all of these problems by simply altering your diet. By eliminating all substances that cause inflammation, your body will begin to flourish. Your epidermis, hair, and nails will become healthier and more robust. You will experience less bloating and less stomach cramping and discomfort. By strengthening your immune system, you will be able to combat disease more effectively. Diet is everything.

How the diet affects inflammation

Utilizing food as medicine to reduce inflammation is one of the most important objectives of the vegan diet. Foods such as unhealthy fats, excessive carbohydrates, processed foods, dairy, and foods of poor quality all cause inflammation in the body. As a result of consuming these foods, insulin levels in the blood rise, which can contribute to insulin resistance, resulting in increased fat storage, inflammation, and immunosuppression.

Leaky intestine is one of the most prevalent inflammatory conditions. Within the digestive system, a cellular lining serves as the adhesive that binds everything together. When this adhesive breaks down, food proteins and bacterial byproducts enter the circulation. When this occurs, you experience an abundance of negative side effects. These effects include skin problems, food sensitivities, and intense fatigue.

This unpleasant health issue is caused by a deficiency of gut flora and an excess of inflammatory foods, which disrupt the delicate gut biome. Leaky gut leads to a dramatic increase in food sensitivities and allergies, which, you guessed it, increases inflammation. Many individuals suffer from leaky intestines without being aware of it.

Eating processed foods containing excessive amounts of carbohydrates, sugar, and wheat will cause inflammation in the body. Particularly, wheat contains gliadins, which are potent pro-inflammatory proteins that disrupt the delicate equilibrium in your gut. This is why many consider wheat to be inflammatory and toxic for digestion.

Focusing on anti-inflammatory nutrients will provide significant mental and physical benefits. More than twenty-five thousand phytochemicals, or plant-derived compounds, are anti-inflammatory. These substances can be found in fruits and vegetables. Spices with anti-inflammatory properties, such as turmeric, rosemary, and ginger, can be readily incorporated into any dish. Vitamin and mineral-rich foods will strengthen your immune system, particularly by preventing inflammation.

Other anti-inflammatory nutrients include those rich in zinc, such as pumpkin seeds and oysters, and Omega-3 fats, such as sardines and herring. Beef liver, cod liver, salmon, and goat cheese all contain Vitamin A, which can repair an imbalanced digestive tract. By introducing beneficial microbes, probiotics in fermented foods such as sauerkraut, pickles, tempeh, miso, and kimchi are also known to promote healthy gut function. Finally, fiber-rich foods such as artichokes, asparagus, plantains, and seaweed will maintain a healthy biome.

Inflammation and an unbalanced microbiome are probable issues that each of us has encountered on occasion. As a result of basing our diets on the recommendations of large corporations and consuming processed wheat and dairy products, our digestive tracts feel terrible and our immune systems are overworked. The vegan diet will enhance digestive health and reduce inflammation.

Increasing Lifespan Through the Pegan Diet

Numerous individuals see their lives ahead of them and wish to extend them whenever conceivable. We all desire to live long, healthy, and fruitful lives in which we spend less time in hospital beds or purchasing medication and more time appreciating all that life has to offer.

The best method to increase our lifespan is to consume a vegan diet. Eating real, whole foods on a vegan diet will turn off the body's inflammatory response, enhance antioxidant systems, and restore hormonal and brain chemistry balance. In addition, it increases your vitality, improves your microbiome, and activates genes that prevent disease. What is there to dislike?

In reality, a large number of prevalent ailments are largely preventable. This knowledge is not taught as frequently as it should be. Typically, organic and natural foods are more expensive than fast cuisine. One method to make a difference is to educate yourself and others on how to prevent disease and illness and increase their lifespan.

Insulin resistance is the underlying cause of heart disease, diabetes, and dementia, among others. In fact, it accelerates muscle wasting with advancing age, resulting in future disability. Insulin resistance occurs when excessive amounts of starch from flour, pasta, bread, rice, and refined cereals are consumed. It also occurs when we consume too much fructose. These nutrients cause the body to produce insulin in order to maintain normal blood sugar levels.

Your body can no longer keep up with you and regulate your blood sugar at some point. This is when type 2 diabetes develops, which is associated with a number of other conditions, including obesity, muscle loss, inflammation, hormonal imbalances, and brain impairment. By resolving the blood-sugar insulin dilemma that so many people contend with unknowingly, you are well on your way to living a long and healthy life.

Pegan for Type 2 Diabetes

Food is a significant cause of chemical imbalances in the body. Dietary changes can resolve insulin resistance and blood sugar regulation issues. Insulin resistance is a pervasive and alarming problem that millions face without their knowledge. By limiting consumption of carbohydrates and sugars, the body will become more balanced over time. The pegan diet is designed to assist individuals with type 2 diabetes or insulin resistance.

Peagan Almond Milk

Ingredients

- 2 dates, pitted
- 1 teaspoon vanilla extract
- 4 cups water, filtered
- 1 cup of almonds, soaked overnight

Instructions

1. First, add the ingredients to a high-speed blender and blend until smooth.

2. Second, pour the liquid into a nut milk bag or piece of cheesecloth to filter.

3. Third, transfer the almond milk to a glass jar or pitcher and refrigerate for two to three hours before serving.

155

Orange And Grapefruit Salad

- 250 g small pink grapefruit
- 16 dried dates
- 250 g small organic orange (1 small organic orange)

1. Rub the orange and grapefruit dry after rinsing them in hot water.
2. Using a sharp knife, thinly peel approx. 3 cm long strip of peel from both fruits and cut into thin strips.
3. Peel the oranges and grapefruits thick enough to remove the white peel.
4. Work on a bowl to collect the juice as you cut the fruit fillets between the separated peels.
5. Divide the dates in half lengthwise, removing the stone as needed and slicing the pulp into very thin strips.
6. In a cup, combine the date strips, fruit fillets, half of the peel strips and the

fresh catch. Allow a steeping period of 15 to 20 minutes.

7. Arrange on a plate and garnish with the remaining strips of peel.

Conclusion

If you adhere to a one-meal-a-day diet, you may be missing out on essential nutrients by avoiding healthful foods such as whole grains, dairy, and beans. Consider flexitarian or Mediterranean diets, which have a more balanced nutritional profile, if you're searching for a healthier eating plan that reduces inflammation.

You may not need to participate in a long-term or short-term diet. But many diets, notably long-term ones, are ineffective. These facts are not endorsements of fad diets or unsustainable weight loss methods, but rather information to help you make an informed decision based on your nutritional requirements, genetic blueprint, budget, and objectives.

If your objective is to lose weight, you can pursue health in numerous other methods. Her primary message is that decreasing weight does not necessarily equate to becoming your healthiest self. Many other lifestyle factors, including exercise, sleep, and nutrition, affect your overall health. Always choose a diet that is balanced and compatible with your lifestyle.

www.ingramcontent.com/pod-product-compliance
Lightning Source LLC
Chambersburg PA
CBHW060504030426
42337CB00015B/1737